The New

Encyclopedia

of Herbal medicine

A Comprehensive Guide on How to Naturally Improve Your Health with Herbs

Noah Emberwood

Introduction

Unlocking the Power of Nature for Health and Well-Being

Welcome to the latest edition of "The New Encyclopedia of Herbal Medicine," your definitive guide to the vast and diverse world of herbal remedies. In these pages, we embark on a journey through centuries of traditional wisdom and cutting-edge research to explore the incredible healing properties of plants that nature has generously bestowed upon us.

Key Features:

1. Comprehensive Herbal Profiles: Dive deep into detailed profiles of a wide array of herbs, each accompanied by historical contexts, traditional uses, and the latest scientific insights into their medicinal potential.

2. Practical Applications: Learn how to harness the therapeutic benefits of herbs in your daily life. Discover effective preparation methods, dosage guidelines, and ways to incorporate herbal remedies into your wellness routine.

3. Evidence-Based Information: Stay informed with evidence-based discussions on the scientific studies supporting the use of herbs for various health conditions. Understand the synergy between traditional knowledge and modern research.

4. Holistic Approach: Embrace a holistic approach to well-being by exploring the interconnectedness of mind, body, and nature. Discover how herbal medicine can complement other wellness practices to foster a balanced and healthy lifestyle.

5. Expert Contributions: Benefit from insights provided by herbalists, naturopaths, and researchers at the forefront of herbal medicine. Their expertise ensures that you receive accurate, up-to-date, and practical information.

"The New Encyclopedia of Herbal Medicine" is more than a reference book; it's a guide to empower you on your journey towards natural health and vitality. Whether you are a seasoned herbal enthusiast or a novice exploring the world of botanicals, this encyclopedia is your trusted companion in unlocking the secrets of herbal medicine.

Herbal wisdom unveiled for holistic health advocates

Herbal wisdom has been an integral part of holistic health practices for centuries, drawing on the healing power of nature to promote well-being and balance in the body, mind, and spirit. Advocates of holistic health recognize the interconnectedness of various aspects of our lives and emphasize the importance of addressing the root causes of imbalances rather than merely treating symptoms. Here are some key aspects of herbal wisdom for holistic health advocates:

1. Plant-Based Healing: Herbal remedies are derived from plants, encompassing leaves, roots, flowers, and seeds. These natural compounds often contain bioactive substances that can have therapeutic effects on the body. Holistic health advocates appreciate the potency of plant-based healing, recognizing that nature provides a rich pharmacy of remedies.

2. Balance and Harmony: Holistic health emphasizes the concept of balance and harmony within the body. Herbs are chosen not just for their symptomatic relief but for their ability to restore equilibrium. Herbal wisdom

encourages a holistic approach that considers physical, emotional, and spiritual well-being as interconnected elements.

3. Preventive Health: Herbal wisdom often involves preventive health measures. Rather than waiting for illness to strike, holistic health advocates integrate herbs into daily routines to support the body's natural defenses and maintain overall health. This proactive approach aligns with the holistic philosophy of nurturing the body's innate ability to heal itself.

4. Individualized Treatment: Holistic health recognizes that each person is unique, and herbal remedies are chosen based on an individual's specific constitution, symptoms, and needs. Herbalists often take into account a person's lifestyle, diet, and emotional well-being to tailor a treatment plan that addresses the root causes of imbalance.

5. Mind-Body Connection: Herbal wisdom acknowledges the intricate connection between the mind and body. Emotional well-being is considered a crucial component of overall health. Certain herbs are chosen for their

calming or uplifting properties, supporting mental and emotional balance alongside physical health.

6. Sustainability: Holistic health advocates are often mindful of sustainability and the impact of their choices on the environment. They may choose herbs that are ethically sourced and promote conservation efforts, recognizing the importance of preserving the delicate balance of ecosystems.

7. Traditional Knowledge and Modern Research: While herbal wisdom draws heavily from traditional knowledge passed down through generations, holistic health advocates also value scientific research. Integrating traditional wisdom with modern evidence-based practices ensures a comprehensive and informed approach to health and wellness.

In embracing herbal wisdom for holistic health, advocates recognize the profound connection between nature and well-being. By incorporating these principles into daily life, individuals can support their health on multiple levels, fostering a sense of balance, resilience, and vitality.

Decoding the secret of Herbal Medicine

Decoding the secrets of herbal medicine involves understanding the intricate relationships between plants and the human body, as well as appreciating the accumulated knowledge passed down through generations. While herbal medicine is often seen as an ancient practice, it continues to be relevant in modern times, with ongoing research providing insights into the mechanisms of action and potential benefits of various herbs. Here are some key aspects to consider when decoding the secrets of herbal medicine:

1. Chemical Complexity: Plants contain a vast array of chemical compounds, including alkaloids, flavonoids, terpenes, and polyphenols, each with unique properties. Decoding herbal medicine involves understanding how these compounds interact with the body at a molecular level, influencing physiological processes and providing therapeutic effects.

2. Synergy and Whole Plant Medicine: The holistic nature of herbal medicine often involves using the whole plant or a combination of plant constituents. The

synergy among different compounds within a plant is believed to enhance therapeutic effects and mitigate potential side effects. Understanding this complexity is crucial for deciphering the secrets of herbal remedies.

3. Traditional Wisdom: Many herbal remedies have been used for centuries in traditional medicine systems worldwide. Decoding herbal medicine requires respecting and understanding the traditional wisdom that has been passed down through generations. This knowledge often includes information on the selection, preparation, and application of herbs for various health conditions.

4. Individualized Treatment: Herbal medicine recognizes that individuals may respond differently to the same herb due to their unique constitution, genetics, and health conditions. Decoding herbal secrets involves tailoring treatments to the individual, considering factors such as lifestyle, diet, and emotional well-being.

5. Adaptogenic Properties: Some herbs are considered adaptogens, helping the body adapt to stressors and maintain balance. Decoding the secrets of adaptogenic

herbs involves understanding their ability to modulate the body's stress response, supporting overall resilience and well-being.

6. Modern Research and Validation: While traditional wisdom forms the foundation of herbal medicine, modern research plays a crucial role in decoding its secrets. Scientific studies help validate traditional uses, identify active compounds, and uncover potential mechanisms of action. Researchers explore the safety and efficacy of herbal remedies through rigorous testing.

7. Bioavailability and Formulation: The way herbs are prepared and consumed can significantly impact their bioavailability—the body's ability to absorb and utilize their active compounds. Decoding herbal medicine involves understanding optimal formulations, such as teas, tinctures, extracts, or capsules, to maximize therapeutic effects.

8. Cultural and Ethical Considerations: Cultural knowledge and ethical sourcing practices contribute to understanding the secrets of herbal medicine. Respecting cultural traditions and ensuring sustainable

harvesting practices help preserve plant diversity and ecosystems.

In essence, decoding the secrets of herbal medicine is a multifaceted process that involves a blend of traditional wisdom, scientific inquiry, and a deep appreciation for the complex interactions between plants and the human body. As research progresses, our understanding of herbal medicine continues to evolve, providing new insights into its potential contributions to holistic health and well-being.

Herbalism Encyclopedia & Apothecary: A Holistic Guide I

Creating a comprehensive herbalism encyclopedia and apothecary guide involves compiling a wealth of information on various herbs, their uses, preparation methods, and therapeutic properties. Such a holistic guide can empower individuals to explore the world of herbal medicine for health and well-being. Here's a suggested outline for your Herbalism Encyclopedia & Apothecary Guide:

Introduction

1. Overview of Herbalism:

   - Definition and principles of herbalism.

   - Historical perspectives on herbal medicine.

   - Modern resurgence and integration with holistic health.

Section 1: Herbal Basics

2. Understanding Herbs:

   - Botanical classifications and plant parts used.

- Herbal actions and energetics.

- The concept of taste in herbalism.

3. Harvesting and Sourcing:

  - Sustainable harvesting practices.

  - Ethical considerations in herb sourcing.

  - Growing your own herbs.

4. Herbal Preparation Methods:

  - Infusions, decoctions, tinctures, poultices, and other preparations.

  - Herbal oil and salve making.

  - Guidelines for proper dosage.

Section 2: Herbal Encyclopedia

5. A-Z Herbal Profiles:

  - In-depth profiles for each herb, including:

    - Botanical name, family, and common names.

    - Historical uses and folklore.

- Constituents and active compounds.

- Therapeutic properties.

- Dosage recommendations and potential contraindications.

- Culinary uses, if applicable.

Section 3: Holistic Health Applications

6. Herbs for Body Systems:

- Herbal support for the respiratory, digestive, circulatory, and nervous systems.

- Adaptogenic herbs for stress and resilience.

- Herbs for immune system support.

7. Herbs for Common Ailments:

- Herbal remedies for headaches, insomnia, digestive issues, etc.

- First aid herbs for minor injuries.

Section 4: Integrating Herbalism into Daily Life

8. Herbal Formulas:

- Recipes for herbal blends targeting specific health goals.

- Creating personalized herbal formulas.

9. Seasonal Herbalism:

- Adapting herbal remedies to different seasons.

- Seasonal foraging and harvesting.

Section 5: Creating an Herbal Apothecary

10. Apothecary Essentials:

- Tools and equipment for herbal preparation.

- Storage and organization of herbs.

- Labeling and record-keeping.

11. Safety and Contraindications:

- Guidelines for safe herbal use.

- Herb-drug interactions.

- Special considerations for pregnancy and children.

Section 6: Resources and Further Learning

12. Books, Websites, and Courses:

 - Recommended reading for beginner and advanced herbalists.

 - Online resources and courses for ongoing learning.

 - Herbal conferences and events.

Conclusion

13. Empowering Holistic Health:

 - Encouragement for readers to explore and integrate herbalism into their lives.

 - Emphasizing the holistic approach to health and well-being.

Remember to regularly update your encyclopedia to include new research findings, emerging herbs, and evolving holistic health practices. Providing clear and concise information will make your guide an invaluable resource for those interested in the world of herbalism.

Herbalism Encyclopedia & Apothecary: A Holistic Guide II

Section 7: Herbal Energetics and Constitutional Medicine

14. Understanding Herbal Energetics:

- Exploring the energetic qualities of herbs (hot, cold, damp, dry).

- Application of herbal energetics in balancing the body.

- Consideration of constitutional types in herbalism.

15. Constitutional Medicine:

- Overview of different constitutional types (e.g., Vata, Pitta, Kapha in Ayurveda).

- Matching herbs to individual constitutions.

- Balancing imbalances through constitutional approaches.

Section 8: Herbal Lore and Folk Medicine

16. Herbal Folklore:

   - Cultural and historical beliefs surrounding herbs.

   - Folk remedies and traditions from various cultures.

   - Superstitions and symbolic meanings associated with herbs.

17. Herbal Rituals and Ceremony:

   - Incorporating herbs into rituals and ceremonies.

   - Herbal cleansing and purification practices.

   - Celebrating seasonal transitions with herbs.

 Section 9: Herbal Entrepreneurship

18. Starting Your Herbal Business:

   - Legal considerations for selling herbal products.

   - Marketing and branding your herbal business.

   - Tips for creating and selling herbal products.

19. Community Engagement:

   - Building a community of herbal enthusiasts.

- Hosting workshops and educational events.

- Collaborating with local businesses and practitioners.

Section 10: Advanced Herbalism

20. Herbal Research and Innovation:

- Current trends in herbal research.

- Innovations in herbal product development.

- The future of herbalism and its potential impact.

21. Herbal Medicine Making Beyond Basics:

- Advanced techniques in herbal extraction.

- Formulating complex herbal remedies.

- Incorporating synergistic herb combinations.

Section 11: Global Herbal Traditions

22. Cross-Cultural Herbalism:

- Exploring herbal traditions from different parts of the world.

- Adapting global herbal practices to local environments.

- Respecting and learning from diverse cultural perspectives.

23. Herbalism in Indigenous Cultures:

- Understanding the importance of cultural sensitivity.

- Preserving and respecting traditional knowledge.

- Supporting indigenous herbal initiatives.

 Section 12: Herbalism and Environmental Stewardship

24. Sustainable Herbalism:

- Ethical wildcrafting and harvesting practices.

- Supporting conservation efforts for endangered plants.

- Cultivating herbs in harmony with the environment.

25. Permaculture and Herbal Gardens:

- Designing herbal gardens based on permaculture principles.

- Creating sustainable and regenerative herbal ecosystems.

- Tips for cultivating herbs at home.

Conclusion

26. Continuing the Herbal Journey:

- Encouraging a lifelong commitment to herbal learning.

- Acknowledging the interconnectedness of herbalism, holistic health, and environmental stewardship.

- Inspiring readers to contribute to the evolving field of herbalism.

By encompassing these additional sections in your Herbalism Encyclopedia & Apothecary Guide, you'll provide a well-rounded resource that caters to various levels of herbal enthusiasts, from beginners to advanced practitioners. The holistic approach ensures a comprehensive understanding of herbalism, incorporating not only the practical aspects but also the cultural, ethical, and environmental dimensions of this ancient healing art.

Native American Herbalism and Alchemy

Native American herbalism and alchemy reflect rich traditions rooted in the intimate connection between indigenous peoples and the natural world. These practices are deeply embedded in spiritual, cultural, and holistic frameworks. Here's an exploration of Native American herbalism and alchemy:

Native American Herbalism:

1. Connection to Nature:

   - Native American herbalism is based on the belief that plants possess spiritual qualities and are interconnected with human well-being.

   - Many tribes view plants as teachers and emphasize the importance of gratitude and reciprocity in harvesting.

2. Sacred Plants:

   - Certain plants hold sacred significance, such as sage, cedar, sweetgrass, and tobacco.

- These sacred plants are often used in ceremonies, rituals, and cleansing practices to purify the mind, body, and spirit.

3. Medicinal Uses:

- Native American herbalists employ a wide variety of plants for medicinal purposes, addressing physical and spiritual aspects of health.

- Examples include yarrow for wound healing, echinacea for immune support, and mullein for respiratory issues.

4. Herbal Rituals:

- Herbalism is intertwined with rituals and ceremonies, involving prayers and offerings to honor the plant spirits.

- The timing of harvest is often guided by lunar cycles, seasonal changes, and specific ceremonies.

5. Healing Wisdom:

- Healing extends beyond the physical, encompassing emotional, mental, and spiritual well-being.

- Native American herbalists often consider the individual's connection to the community and the land in their healing practices.

6. Intergenerational Knowledge:

- Herbal knowledge is passed down through generations within tribes, fostering a deep sense of cultural continuity.

- Elders and medicine people play crucial roles in preserving and transmitting herbal wisdom.

Native American Alchemy:

1. Spiritual Alchemy:

- Native American alchemy is rooted in spiritual transformation and the transmutation of the self.

- Rituals, vision quests, and ceremonial practices are forms of alchemical processes aimed at personal growth and enlightenment.

2. Symbolism in Art and Crafts:

- Native American art often incorporates alchemical symbols representing transformation, balance, and the interconnectedness of all things.

- Crafts, such as pottery and jewelry, may hold symbolic meanings related to alchemical principles.

3. Alchemy in Symbolic Stories:

- Traditional stories and myths convey alchemical principles, representing the journey of self-discovery, balance, and transformation.

- Animal symbolism often plays a role in conveying alchemical wisdom.

4. Alchemy of Plants and Elements:

- Native American alchemy acknowledges the transformative power of plants and elements, seeing them as agents of change and healing.

- The balance and harmony of the natural world are considered essential aspects of alchemical processes.

5. Ceremonial Alchemy:

- Ceremonies, dances, and rituals are seen as alchemical processes that connect individuals to the spiritual realm and facilitate personal transformation.

- Sweat lodges and vision quests are examples of ceremonies with alchemical significance.

Integration of Herbalism and Alchemy:

1. Energetic Healing:

- Both herbalism and alchemy within Native American traditions often focus on balancing and harmonizing the energetic aspects of the individual.

2. Ceremonial Herbs:

- The use of ceremonial herbs, such as sage and sweetgrass, exemplifies the integration of herbalism into alchemical and spiritual practices.

3. Sacred Spaces:

- Creating sacred spaces using herbs and elements contributes to the alchemical environment, supporting transformation and spiritual growth.

4. Balance and Harmony:

 - The holistic approach of Native American herbalism and alchemy emphasizes the importance of balance and harmony within oneself and the broader natural world.

In summary, Native American herbalism and alchemy are deeply intertwined practices that encompass healing, spirituality, and personal transformation. These traditions offer profound insights into the interconnectedness of humans and the natural world, emphasizing the importance of maintaining harmony for overall well-being.

Essence of Essential Oils

Essential oils are concentrated plant extracts that capture the aromatic and therapeutic essence of a plant. These oils are extracted from various parts of plants, including leaves, flowers, bark, stems, and roots. Here's a closer look at the essence of essential oils:

1. Extraction Methods:

   - Distillation: The most common method, where steam is used to extract the essential oil from the plant material.

   - Expression or Cold-Pressing: Typically used for citrus oils, where mechanical pressure is applied to release the oil.

   - Solvent Extraction: Involves using a solvent to extract the oil; the solvent is then evaporated to leave behind the essential oil.

2. Chemical Composition:

   - Volatile Compounds: Essential oils are rich in volatile compounds that give them their characteristic aroma.

- Terpenes: A large group of compounds found in essential oils with diverse therapeutic properties.

- Phenols, Aldehydes, Esters, and Oxides: Different chemical classes contribute to the unique properties of each essential oil.

3. Aromatic Properties:

- Fragrance Profiles: Essential oils have a wide range of fragrances, from floral and citrusy to earthy and spicy.

- Therapeutic Aromatherapy: Aromatherapists use essential oils to influence mood, emotions, and cognitive function through inhalation.

4. Therapeutic Benefits:

- Antimicrobial Properties: Many essential oils have natural antimicrobial and antibacterial properties.

- Anti-Inflammatory Effects: Some oils exhibit anti-inflammatory properties, making them useful in skincare and pain relief.

- Relaxation and Stress Relief: Certain essential oils, like lavender and chamomile, are known for their calming effects on the nervous system.

5. Application Methods:

- Topical Application: Diluted essential oils can be applied to the skin for various purposes, such as massage or skincare.

- Inhalation: Diffusing oils in the air or inhaling directly from the bottle can provide therapeutic benefits.

- Internal Use (with Caution): Some essential oils are considered safe for internal use but should be used cautiously and with proper guidance.

6. Carrier Oils:

- Essential oils are often diluted in carrier oils before topical application to reduce the risk of irritation.

- Common carrier oils include jojoba, coconut, almond, and olive oil.

7. Safety Considerations:

- Skin Sensitivity: Some essential oils can cause skin irritation, so they should be diluted before use.

- Phototoxicity: Certain citrus oils can make the skin more sensitive to sunlight.

- Pregnancy and Children: Pregnant women and young children may need to avoid or use certain oils cautiously.

8. Popular Essential Oils:

- Lavender: Calming and versatile, used for relaxation and skincare.

- Peppermint: Energizing and invigorating, often used for headaches and digestion.

- Tea Tree: Antimicrobial and anti-inflammatory, commonly used for skin issues.

- Eucalyptus: Respiratory support, helpful for congestion and colds.

9. Quality and Purity:

- Therapeutic-Grade Oils: Look for oils that are labeled as pure and free from additives.

- Sourcing: High-quality oils are often sourced from reputable suppliers and sustainable practices.

10. Culinary Uses:

- Some essential oils are safe for consumption and can be used in cooking to add flavor to dishes.

11. Holistic Wellness:

- Essential oils are often embraced in holistic wellness practices for their physical, emotional, and spiritual benefits.

Understanding the essence of essential oils involves recognizing their chemical complexity, therapeutic potential, and diverse applications. When used mindfully and with respect for safety considerations, essential oils can enhance well-being and contribute to holistic health practices.

Herbal Remedies Unveiled

Herbal remedies have been used for centuries across various cultures for their potential health benefits. Unveiling the secrets of herbal remedies involves understanding the properties of specific plants and how they can be harnessed for various health concerns. Here's a glimpse into the world of herbal remedies:

1. Holistic Approach:

- Herbal remedies often embrace a holistic approach, considering the interconnectedness of the body, mind, and spirit.

- The goal is not just to treat symptoms but to address the root causes of imbalances in the body.

2. Common Herbal Remedies:

- Echinacea: Known for immune system support, particularly during cold and flu seasons.

- Chamomile: Valued for its calming properties, often used for stress and sleep-related issues.

- Ginger: A popular remedy for digestive issues, nausea, and inflammation.

- Turmeric: Recognized for its anti-inflammatory and antioxidant properties.

- Peppermint: Used for digestive relief and to soothe headaches.

3. Adaptogenic Herbs:

- Ashwagandha: An adaptogen known for its ability to help the body adapt to stress and promote overall well-being.

- Rhodiola: Another adaptogen believed to enhance resilience to stress.

4. Herbs for Sleep:

- Valerian: Commonly used as a natural remedy for sleep disorders and insomnia.

- Lavender: Known for its calming aroma, often used to promote relaxation and improve sleep.

5. Anti-Anxiety Herbs:

- Passionflower: Used to alleviate symptoms of anxiety and promote relaxation.

- Kava Kava: Traditionally used in the South Pacific for its calming effects.

6. Herbs for Skin Health:

- Calendula: Applied topically for its soothing properties on the skin.

- Aloe Vera: Known for its cooling and healing effects on the skin.

7. Herbs for Respiratory Health:

- Thyme: Recognized for its antibacterial properties, often used for respiratory issues.

- Licorice Root: Known for its soothing effects on the throat and respiratory system.

8. Traditional Herbal Systems:

- Ayurveda: Incorporates herbs like holy basil (Tulsi), triphala, and ashwagandha for holistic well-being.

- Traditional Chinese Medicine (TCM): Utilizes herbs like ginseng, astragalus, and goji berries for balancing the body's vital energy (Qi).

9. Herbal Teas:

- Many herbs are consumed in the form of teas for their soothing and therapeutic effects.

- Examples include chamomile tea, peppermint tea, and ginger tea.

10. Dosage and Preparation:

- Herbal remedies can be prepared in various forms, including teas, tinctures, capsules, and salves.

- Proper dosage and preparation methods are crucial for safety and effectiveness.

11. Scientific Research:

- Ongoing scientific studies explore the efficacy and safety of herbal remedies.

- Research contributes to a better understanding of the mechanisms behind the therapeutic properties of certain herbs.

12. Individualized Approaches:

- Effective herbal remedies often consider individual differences, such as constitution, lifestyle, and existing health conditions.

- Consulting with a qualified herbalist can help tailor remedies to individual needs.

13. Safety Considerations:

- While many herbs are safe, it's essential to be aware of potential interactions and contraindications.

- Pregnant and nursing individuals should exercise caution and seek professional guidance.

14. Cultural Wisdom:

- Herbal remedies often draw from cultural traditions and indigenous knowledge passed down through generations.

- Respecting and understanding these cultural perspectives enhances the efficacy of herbal practices.

15. Sustainable Harvesting:

- Emphasizing sustainable harvesting practices helps preserve the biodiversity of medicinal plants and supports environmental stewardship.

Unveiling the potential of herbal remedies involves a combination of traditional wisdom, scientific inquiry, and a holistic understanding of health and well-being. Integrating these remedies into a balanced lifestyle can contribute to a more natural and holistic approach to self-care. It's important to approach herbal remedies with respect, knowledge, and an awareness of individual health needs.

A Natural Approach to Common Ailments

A natural approach to common ailments involves harnessing the healing power of nature to support the body's innate ability to restore balance and well-being. Here's a guide to addressing some common ailments through natural means:

1. Colds and Flu:

- Herbal Teas: Ginger, elderberry, echinacea, and peppermint teas can provide relief and boost the immune system.

- Hydration: Drink plenty of fluids like warm water with lemon, herbal teas, and broths.

- Rest: Allow the body to rest and recover.

2. Digestive Issues:

- Peppermint Oil: Helps alleviate symptoms of indigestion and bloating.

- Ginger Tea: Aids digestion and relieves nausea.

- Probiotics: Consume fermented foods like yogurt or kefir to promote gut health.

3. Headaches:

- Hydration: Dehydration can contribute to headaches; drink water throughout the day.

- Peppermint Oil: Apply diluted peppermint oil to temples for a cooling effect.

- Relaxation Techniques: Practice deep breathing or meditation to reduce stress-related headaches.

4. Stress and Anxiety:

- Herbal Teas: Chamomile, passionflower, and valerian root teas have calming properties.

- Aromatherapy: Lavender, bergamot, and frankincense essential oils can be diffused or applied topically for relaxation.

- Exercise: Regular physical activity can help manage stress.

5. Insomnia:

- Valerian Root Tea: Known for its calming effects on the nervous system.

- Lavender Oil: Diffuse or apply diluted lavender oil for its sleep-inducing properties.

- Establish a Routine: Create a consistent sleep schedule and practice relaxation before bedtime.

6. Skin Irritations:

- Aloe Vera Gel: Soothes sunburns, insect bites, and minor skin irritations.

- Calendula Cream: Has anti-inflammatory properties and is beneficial for dry or irritated skin.

- Tea Tree Oil: Diluted tea tree oil can be applied topically for its antimicrobial properties.

7. Muscle Pain and Joint Discomfort:

- Arnica Gel or Cream: Applied topically for relieving muscle soreness.

- Epsom Salt Bath: Soaking in an Epsom salt bath can help relax muscles and reduce inflammation.

- Turmeric Supplements: Known for its anti-inflammatory properties; consult a healthcare professional for guidance.

8. Allergies:

- Quercetin-Rich Foods: Apples, berries, and onions contain quercetin, which may help manage allergies.

- Local Honey: Consuming local honey may help build tolerance to local pollen.

- Nettle Tea: Known for its antihistamine properties.

9. Menstrual Cramps:

- Ginger Tea: Known for its anti-inflammatory and pain-relieving properties.

- Heat Therapy: Applying a heating pad to the lower abdomen can provide relief.

- Dietary Changes: Consuming magnesium-rich foods may help alleviate cramps.

10. Earaches:

- Garlic Oil Drops: Natural antimicrobial properties may help with ear infections.

- Warm Compress: Applying a warm compress to the affected ear can provide relief.

- Chiropractic Care: Gentle adjustments may help with ear-related issues; consult a healthcare professional.

General Tips:

- Stay Hydrated: Proper hydration supports overall health and aids in the body's natural healing processes.

- Nutrient-Rich Diet: Focus on a diet rich in fruits, vegetables, whole grains, and lean proteins to provide essential nutrients.

- Regular Exercise: Physical activity supports overall well-being and can help manage stress.

- Mind-Body Practices: Incorporate practices like meditation, yoga, or deep breathing to promote holistic health.

It's important to note that while natural approaches can be beneficial for many individuals, it's crucial to consult with healthcare professionals, especially in cases of chronic or severe conditions. Integrating these natural strategies with personalized medical advice can contribute to a holistic approach to health and well-being.

Crafting Herbal Magic: Recipes for Wellness

"Crafting Herbal Magic: Recipes for Wellness" invites you to explore the enchanting world of herbal remedies, where the magic of nature meets the art of healing. From soothing teas to invigorating salves, these recipes are crafted with intention to promote holistic wellness and balance. Here's a collection of magical herbal recipes for your well-being:

1. Elixir of Vitality:

   - Ingredients:

     - 1 tsp elderberry syrup

     - 1 tbsp rosehip powder

     - 1/2 tsp astragalus root powder

     - 1 cup hot water

   - Instructions:

     1. Mix ingredients in hot water.

     2. Infuse with intentions for vitality and immune support.

3. Sip slowly and visualize your body thriving with energy.

2. Dreamweaver Tea:

  - Ingredients:

    - 1 tsp dried lavender

    - 1 tsp chamomile flowers

    - 1 tsp lemon balm

    - 1 cup hot water

  - Instructions:

    1. Steep herbs in hot water.

    2. Enchant the tea with dreams of peaceful sleep.

    3. Drink before bedtime for restful and magical dreams.

3. Tranquil Tincture:

  - Ingredients:

    - 1 oz passionflower tincture

    - 1 oz valerian root tincture

    - 1 oz chamomile tincture

- Instructions:

  1. Blend tinctures in equal parts.

  2. Charge with calming energy and intentions.

  3. Take a few drops before bedtime for tranquil nights.

4. Glowing Goddess Face Mask:

 - Ingredients:

   - 2 tbsp honey

   - 1 tbsp powdered turmeric

   - 1 tsp rosewater

 - Instructions:

   1. Mix ingredients to form a paste.

   2. Apply to the face, infusing the mask with self-love.

   3. Relax for 15 minutes before gently rinsing off.

5. Joyful Heart Elixir:

 - Ingredients:

   - 1 oz hawthorn berry tincture

   - 1 oz rose petal tincture

- 1 oz motherwort tincture

- Instructions:

1. Combine tinctures with loving intentions.

2. In times of emotional need, take a few drops to uplift the heart.

6. Herbal Energy Spell Oil:

- Ingredients:

- 1/2 cup jojoba oil

- 7 drops peppermint essential oil

- 5 drops rosemary essential oil

- A pinch of dried basil

- Instructions:

1. Mix oils and herbs in a glass bottle.

2. Charge the blend with energy for focus and vitality.

3. Anoint pulse points when needing an energy boost.

7. Serenity Bath Salts:

- Ingredients:

- 1 cup Epsom salt

- 1/2 cup dried lavender buds

- 10 drops lavender essential oil

- Instructions:

1. Combine ingredients and charge with serenity.

2. Add to a warm bath to soak away stress and tension.

8. Empowerment Herbal Smoke Blend:

- Ingredients:

- 1 part mugwort

- 1 part damiana

- 1 part rosemary

- Instructions:

1. Blend herbs with intentions of empowerment.

2. Burn in a fireproof vessel, visualizing strength and courage.

9. Grounding Forest Infusion:

- Ingredients:

- 1 tbsp pine needles

- 1 tbsp nettle leaves

- 1 tbsp oat straw

- 1 cup hot water

- Instructions:

1. Steep herbs in hot water.

2. Connect with the grounding energy of the forest.

3. Drink mindfully for a rooted sense of balance.

10. Prosperity Potion:

 - Ingredients:

- 1 cinnamon stick

- 3 whole cloves

- 1 slice of fresh ginger

- 1 cup hot water

- Instructions:

1. Infuse hot water with the spices.

2. Stir clockwise, focusing on abundance and prosperity.

3. Sip slowly, embracing the energy of prosperity.

Craft these herbal wonders with mindfulness and intention, letting the magic of herbs enhance your well-being on all levels—physical, emotional, and spiritual. May these recipes bring healing and enchantment to your wellness journey.

Herbal Remedies for the Little Ones

Herbal remedies can be gentle and effective options for supporting the health and well-being of little ones. However, it's essential to use caution, and it's recommended to consult with a pediatrician or a qualified herbalist before introducing herbal remedies to children. Here are some herbal remedies suitable for children, keeping in mind their safety and potential effectiveness:

1. Chamomile Tea for Digestive Comfort:

  - Ingredients:

    - 1 teaspoon dried chamomile flowers

    - 1 cup hot water

  - Instructions:

    1. Steep chamomile flowers in hot water.

    2. Allow the tea to cool to a safe temperature.

    3. Offer small sips for relief from indigestion or to promote relaxation.

2. Honey and Lemon for Cough:

 - Ingredients:

   - 1 teaspoon raw honey

   - A few drops of fresh lemon juice

 - Instructions:

   1. Mix honey and lemon in a spoon.

   2. Give a small amount to soothe a cough (for children over one year old).

3. Calendula Salve for Skin Irritations:

 - Ingredients:

   - Calendula-infused oil

   - Beeswax (for consistency)

 - Instructions:

   1. Mix calendula oil with melted beeswax.

   2. Apply the salve to minor cuts, scrapes, or skin irritations.

4. Ginger and Peppermint Tea for Nausea:

 - Ingredients:

- Fresh ginger slices

- Peppermint leaves

- 1 cup hot water

- Instructions:

1. Steep ginger slices and peppermint leaves in hot water.

2. Offer the tea at a mild temperature to alleviate nausea.

5. Lavender Sachet for Sleep:

- Ingredients:

- Dried lavender flowers

- Small cotton sachet bag

- Instructions:

1. Place dried lavender flowers in the sachet bag.

2. Place the sachet near the child's pillow to promote restful sleep.

6. Fennel Seed Infusion for Colic:

- Ingredients:

- 1 teaspoon fennel seeds

- 1 cup hot water

- Instructions:

1. Steep fennel seeds in hot water.

2. Offer a small amount for infants experiencing colic.

7. Echinacea Popsicles for Immune Support:

- Ingredients:

- Echinacea tea (cooled)

- Unsweetened fruit juice

- Instructions:

1. Mix cooled echinacea tea with fruit juice.

2. Freeze the mixture in popsicle molds for a tasty immune boost.

8. Oatmeal Bath for Eczema or Skin Irritation:

- Ingredients:

- Colloidal oatmeal

- Warm bathwater

- Instructions:

1. Add colloidal oatmeal to warm bathwater.

2. Allow the child to soak for relief from eczema or irritated skin.

9. Peppermint Oil Inhalation for Congestion (Age-Appropriate):

  - Ingredients:

    - 1 drop peppermint essential oil

    - Diffuser or bowl of hot water

  - Instructions:

1. Use a diffuser or place a bowl of hot water with a drop of peppermint oil in the child's room to ease congestion (for children over six years old).

10. Nettle Leaf Infusion for Allergies:

  - Ingredients:

    - 1 teaspoon dried nettle leaves

    - 1 cup hot water

  - Instructions:

1. Steep nettle leaves in hot water.

2. Offer the child a small amount to help manage allergies.

Important Considerations:

- Dosage: Always follow recommended dosages for herbal remedies, and adjust based on the child's age and weight.

- Consultation: Seek advice from a healthcare professional or qualified herbalist before introducing new herbs or remedies.

- Age Appropriateness: Some herbs may not be suitable for very young children, so it's crucial to choose age-appropriate remedies.

Remember, each child is unique, and what works for one may not work for another. Be observant of any allergic reactions or adverse effects, and discontinue use if needed. The goal is to use herbal remedies safely and effectively to enhance the well-being of your little ones.

Native American at Home - A DIY Herbal Adventure

Embarking on a DIY herbal adventure inspired by Native American traditions can be a beautiful way to connect with nature, promote well-being, and honor indigenous wisdom. Here's a guide for creating your Native American-inspired herbal at-home experience:

1. Herb Gathering Ritual:

   - Intentions: Set positive intentions for your herbal adventure, focusing on gratitude, respect for nature, and connection with the plant spirits.

   - Sacred Space: Create a sacred space in your home using symbolic elements like feathers, stones, or native artwork.

   - Herb Gathering: If possible, gather herbs from your local area respectfully, or source them from a trusted supplier.

2. DIY Herbal Smudge Sticks:

   - Ingredients:

- Sage, cedar, sweetgrass, lavender, or other dried herbs.

   - Cotton or hemp twine.

 - Instructions:

   1. Bundle the herbs together and tie them with twine.

   2. Allow the bundle to dry completely.

   3. Use your homemade smudge stick for purification rituals or to cleanse your space.

3. Medicinal Tea Blending:

  - Native Plants: Explore native plants like yarrow, mint, goldenrod, or echinacea.

  - Blending Ritual: Intuitively blend herbs, focusing on their medicinal properties and your wellness intentions.

  - Brewing Ceremony: Brew your tea mindfully, embracing the medicinal qualities of each herb.

4. Herbal Dream Pillows:

  - Ingredients:

   - Lavender, mugwort, hops, or other dream-enhancing herbs.

- Fabric and thread for the pillow.

 - Instructions:

   1. Create a small pillow filled with dream herbs.

   2. Place it under your regular pillow to enhance dreams and encourage restful sleep.

5. DIY Herbal Infused Oil:

  - Ingredients:

    - Calendula flowers, chamomile, or plantain.

    - Carrier oil (such as olive or jojoba).

  - Instructions:

   1. Combine herbs and carrier oil in a glass jar.

   2. Allow it to infuse in a sunny spot for a few weeks.

   3. Strain and use the infused oil for massages or skincare.

 6. Herbal Storytelling:

  - Plant Spirit Communication: Sit with your chosen herbs and meditate on their energies.

- Create a Story: Develop a short story or poem that honors the spirit of the plants and your connection to them.

- Share the Tale: Share your herbal story with others or keep it as a personal reflection.

7. Herbal Art and Craft:

- Nature Printing: Use leaves and flowers to create beautiful prints on paper or fabric.

- Herbal Dyeing: Explore natural dyeing with plants like turmeric, elderberry, or onion skins.

- Herbal Mandala: Arrange dried herbs into a mandala, expressing gratitude for each plant's unique energy.

8. Herbal Bath Ritual:

- Ingredients:

  - Dried herbs like chamomile, rose petals, or lavender.

  - Epsom salt.

- Instructions:

1. Mix herbs and Epsom salt in a sachet or directly into your bath.

2. Soak in the herbal-infused water, allowing the plants to rejuvenate your body and spirit.

9. Herbal Offerings and Gratitude:

- Offerings: Create small bundles of herbs as offerings to express gratitude for the plant spirits.

- Outdoor Ceremony: If possible, perform a simple ceremony outdoors, acknowledging the land and giving thanks.

10. Herbal Wisdom Journaling:

- Reflective Writing: Journal your experiences, thoughts, and insights gained during your herbal adventure.

- Future Intentions: Set intentions for continued connection with herbal wisdom and nature.

Remember to approach your DIY herbal adventure with reverence, respect, and a willingness to learn. Connect with the plants with a humble heart, acknowledging the rich traditions and wisdom of Native American herbal practices.

Conclusion

Embarking on a Native American-inspired DIY herbal adventure offers a meaningful journey into the rich tapestry of indigenous wisdom, connecting us with nature's healing energies. As we conclude this exploration, let us reflect on the key themes and takeaways:

1. Cultural Respect:

   - Approach the herbal adventure with deep respect for Native American traditions. Acknowledge the cultural significance of the practices and honor the wisdom passed down through generations.

2. Connection with Nature:

   - Foster a genuine connection with nature by gathering herbs mindfully and with gratitude. Embrace the idea that plants have spirits and offer their wisdom for our well-being.

3. Sacred Rituals:

- Create sacred spaces and engage in rituals with intention. Whether crafting herbal smudge sticks, blending teas, or infusing oils, infuse each step with a sense of reverence and purpose.

4. Mindful Crafting:

- The DIY herbal creations, from smudge sticks to dream pillows, become more than mere crafts; they become conduits for spiritual and medicinal energies. Approach each creation as a work of art and a reflection of your connection with the natural world.

5. Spiritual Awareness:

- Cultivate spiritual awareness by engaging in practices like herbal storytelling, where the spirit of plants is celebrated. Use your herbal adventure as an opportunity for self-reflection and a deeper understanding of the interconnectedness of all living beings.

6. Holistic Wellness:

- Embrace the holistic approach to wellness by blending medicinal teas, creating herbal-infused oils, and incorporating herbs into bath rituals. Recognize that well-being encompasses the physical, emotional, and spiritual aspects of our being.

7. Gratitude and Offerings:

   - Express gratitude for the gifts of the land and acknowledge the plant spirits through offerings. This practice deepens the sense of reciprocity and respect within the herbal journey.

8. Creative Expression:

   - Engage in creative expressions like nature printing, herbal dyeing, and crafting mandalas. Allow your creativity to flow, guided by the energies of the plants and the inspiration drawn from Native American traditions.

9. Continued Learning:

   - Recognize that the herbal adventure is an ongoing process of learning and growth. Continue to explore, research, and expand your knowledge of Native American herbalism while respecting the diversity of indigenous traditions.

10. Personal Reflection:

- Journal your experiences, insights, and the spiritual connections forged during the herbal adventure. Use your reflections to deepen your understanding of the plants and their role in your personal journey.

In conclusion, the DIY herbal adventure inspired by Native American traditions offers a holistic and transformative experience. As you engage in this exploration, may you find balance, healing, and a profound sense of connection with the natural world and its sacred teachings. May your herbal journey be a tapestry woven with threads of respect, gratitude, and the enduring wisdom of indigenous cultures.

www.ingramcontent.com/pod-product-compliance
Lightning Source LLC
Chambersburg PA
CBHW071101260726

48661CB00006B/2385